I0753834

# SIMON the SCARED ROTTWEILER

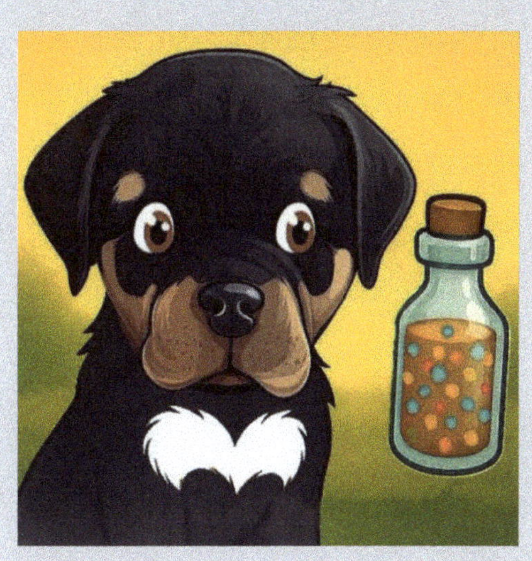

NICOLE S. KLUEMPER, Ph.D.

# Simon the Scared Rottweiler



ISBN: 979-8-218-88480-2

Published by Nicole S. Kluemper, Ph.D., La Mesa, California 91941

Printed in the United States of America.



PUBLISHER'S NOTE: This book is a work of fiction. Names, characters, places, and incidents are either the product of the author's imagination or are used fictitiously.

Author and owner of illustrations: Nicole S. Klumper, Ph.D.

Luanna K. Leisure, Little White Feather Graphic Artist and Independent Publisher, Campbell, California 95008. www.luannaleisurebooks.com.

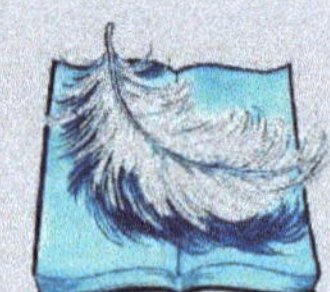

To order additional books go to: www.lulu.com, Amazon.com, and other online bookstores.
Website: www.nicolekluemper.com
Email: simonthescaredrottweiler@gmail.com

Appendix: Page 25-26. How to make a thought bottle with belly breathing instructions and contact information on national child anxiety and crisis resources.

Dedicated to all the Rottweilers I've loved.
You made me a better person. Thank you.

Nicole

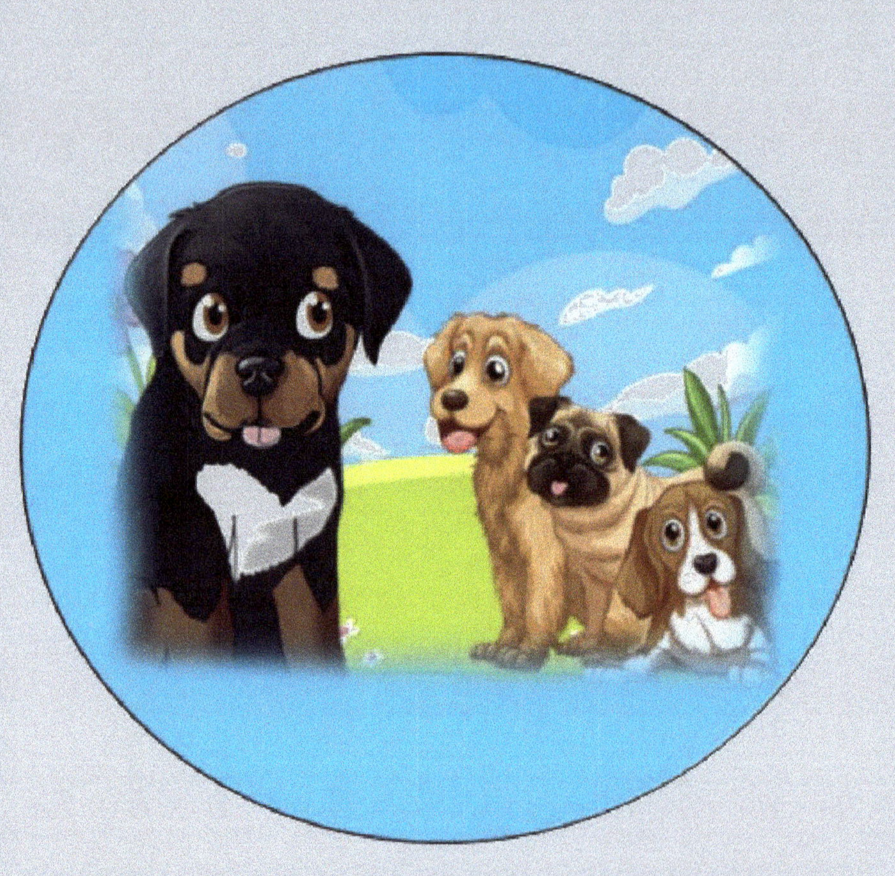

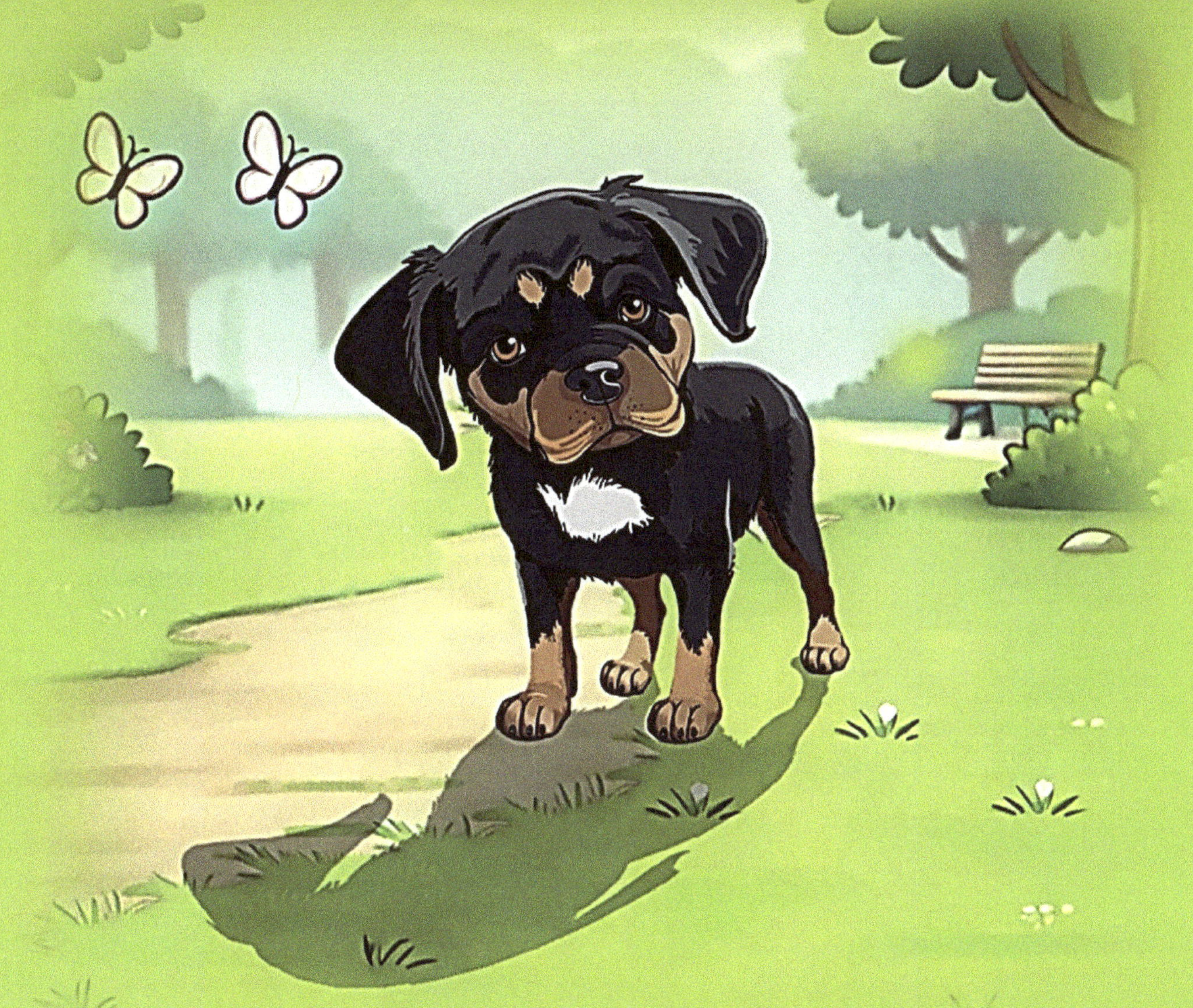

My name is Simon. Even though I'm a Rottweiler, and people are usually scared of me, I get scared sometimes too. A few weeks ago, I had a really scary day.

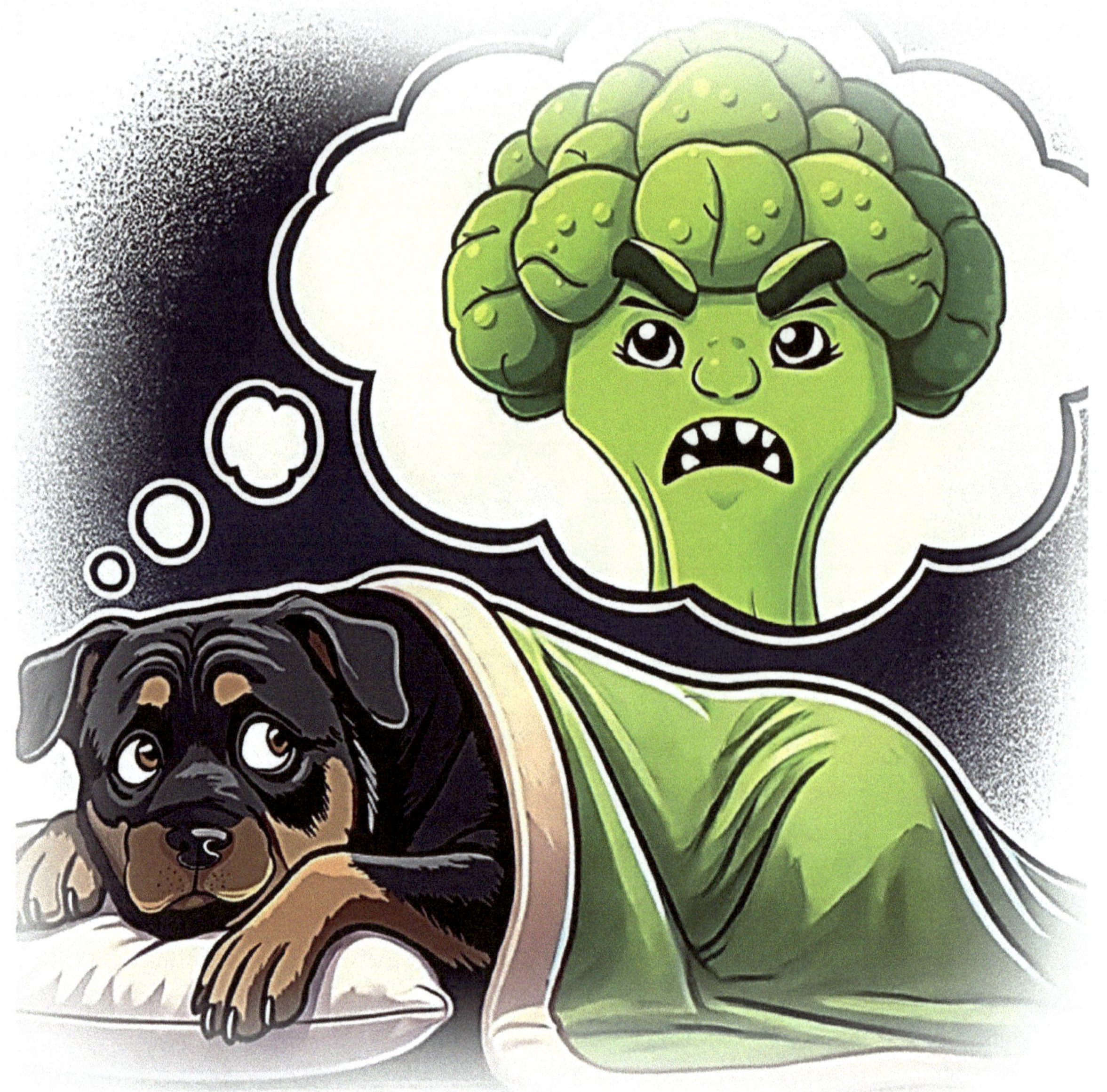

I woke up to a really bad dream – I was being chased by a huge piece of broccoli! I don't know about you, but it doesn't get any scarier than that for me.

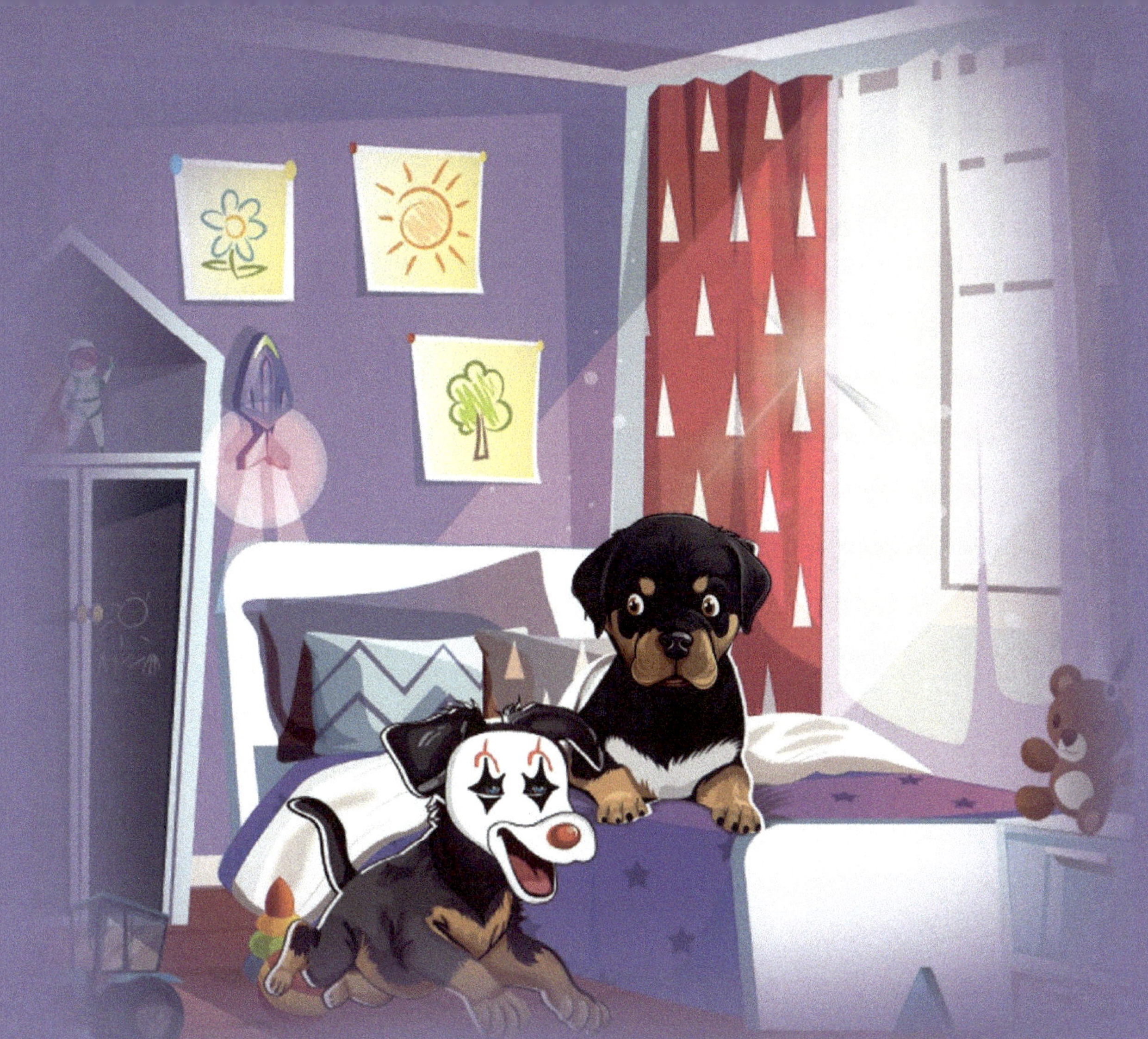

I got up and went looking for Mom, and my brother jumped out from under the bed with a clown mask on! He scared me really bad!! I told him I didn't think he was funny, but he just laughed and laughed.

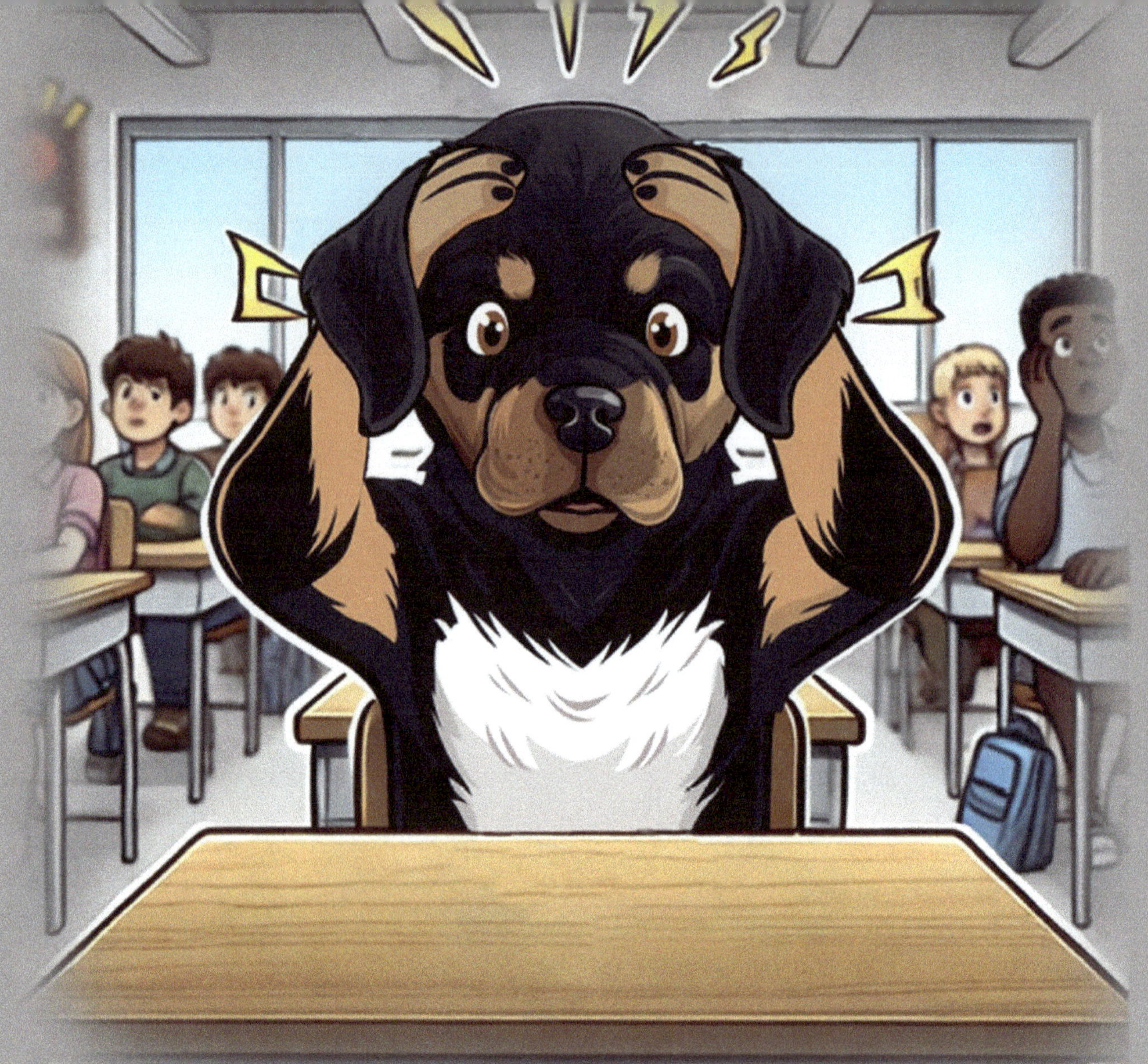

I was sitting in English class when all of a sudden, the fire alarm went off. Not only did it surprise me, but I didn't know whether it was real or not, and I was scared.

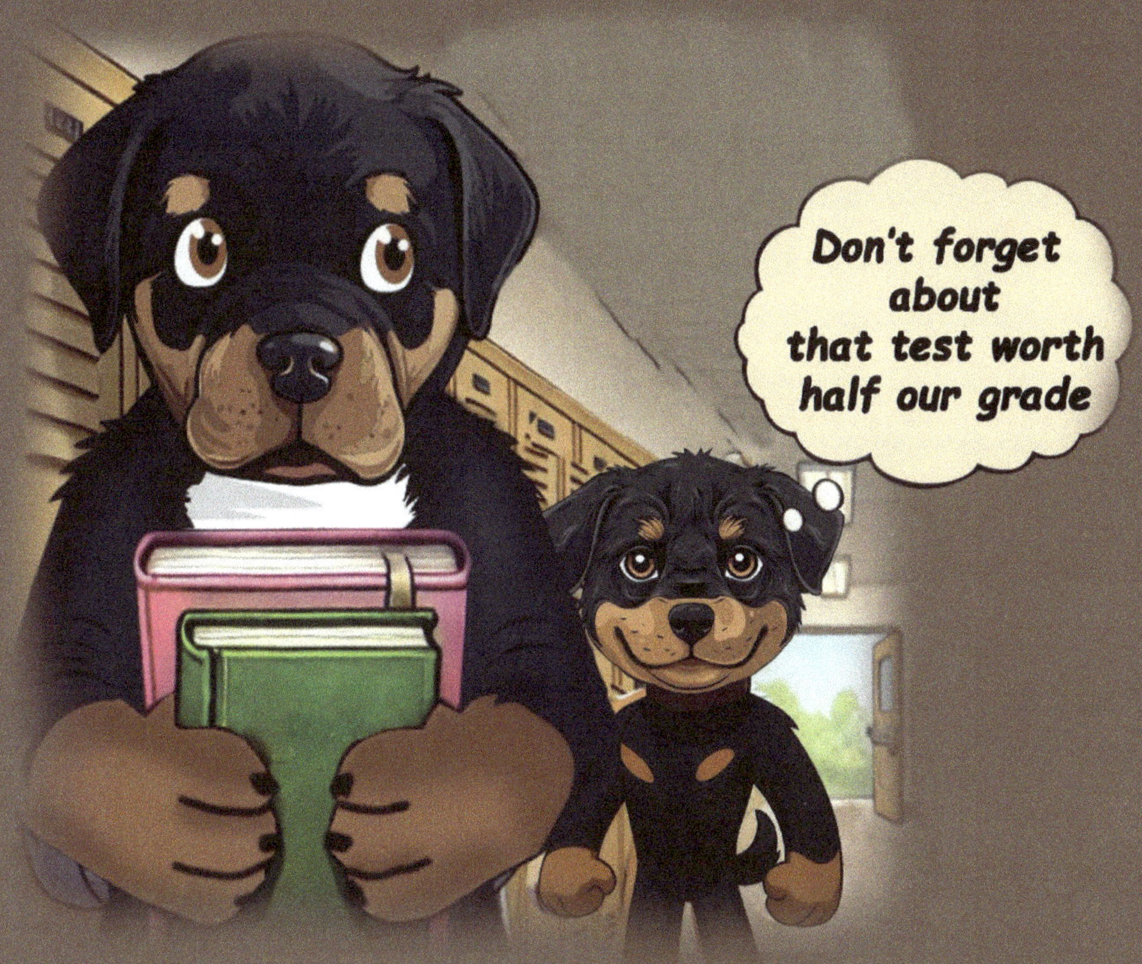


Right before math class, my friend Kevin reminded me that we had a huge test that was worth almost half our grade! I thought I was going to lose my breakfast I was so nervous.

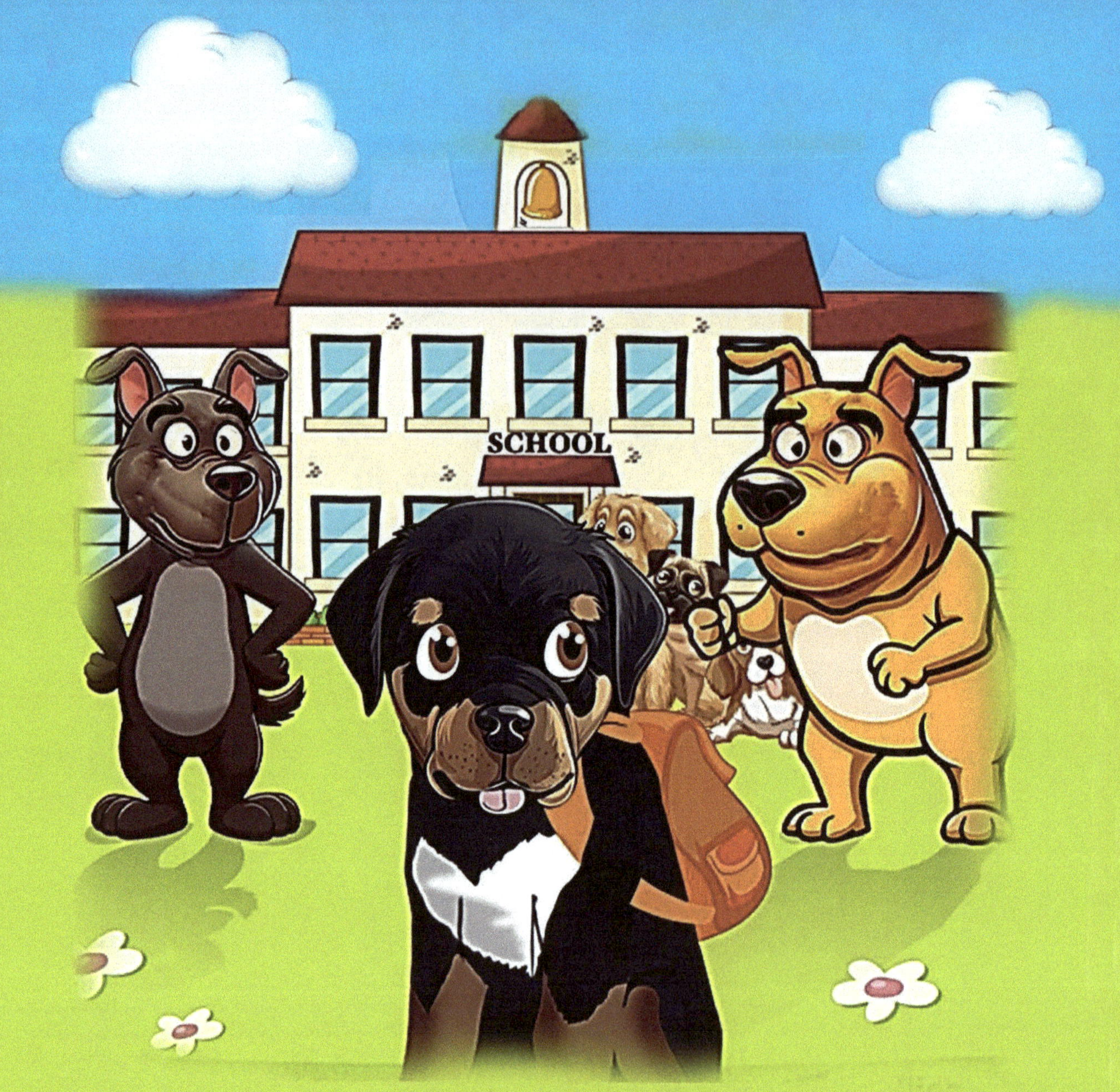


Finally, I made it to after school, and some big bullies tried to mess with me and my friends.

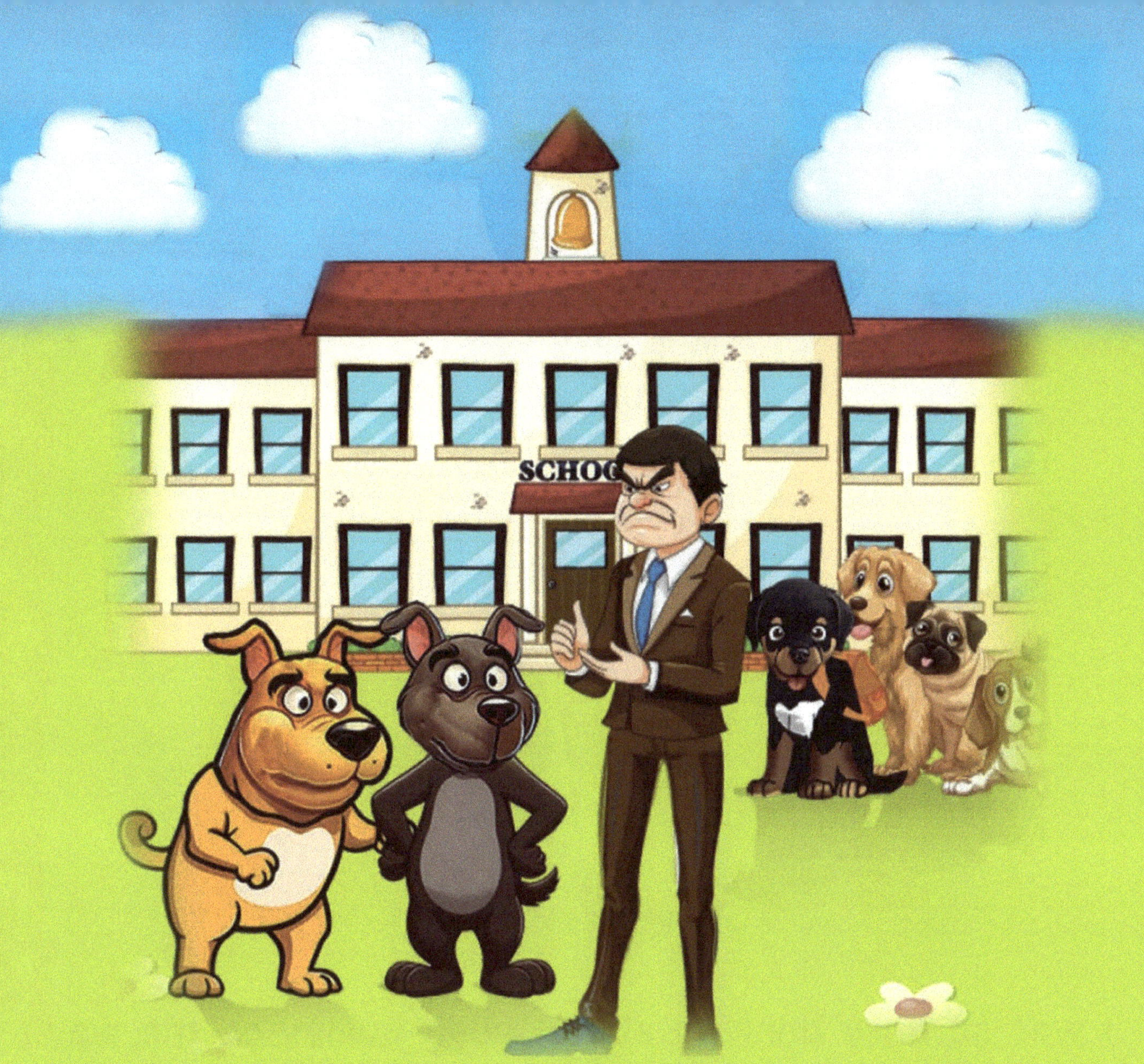

Just when I thought we were done for, the principal showed up. Thank goodness!

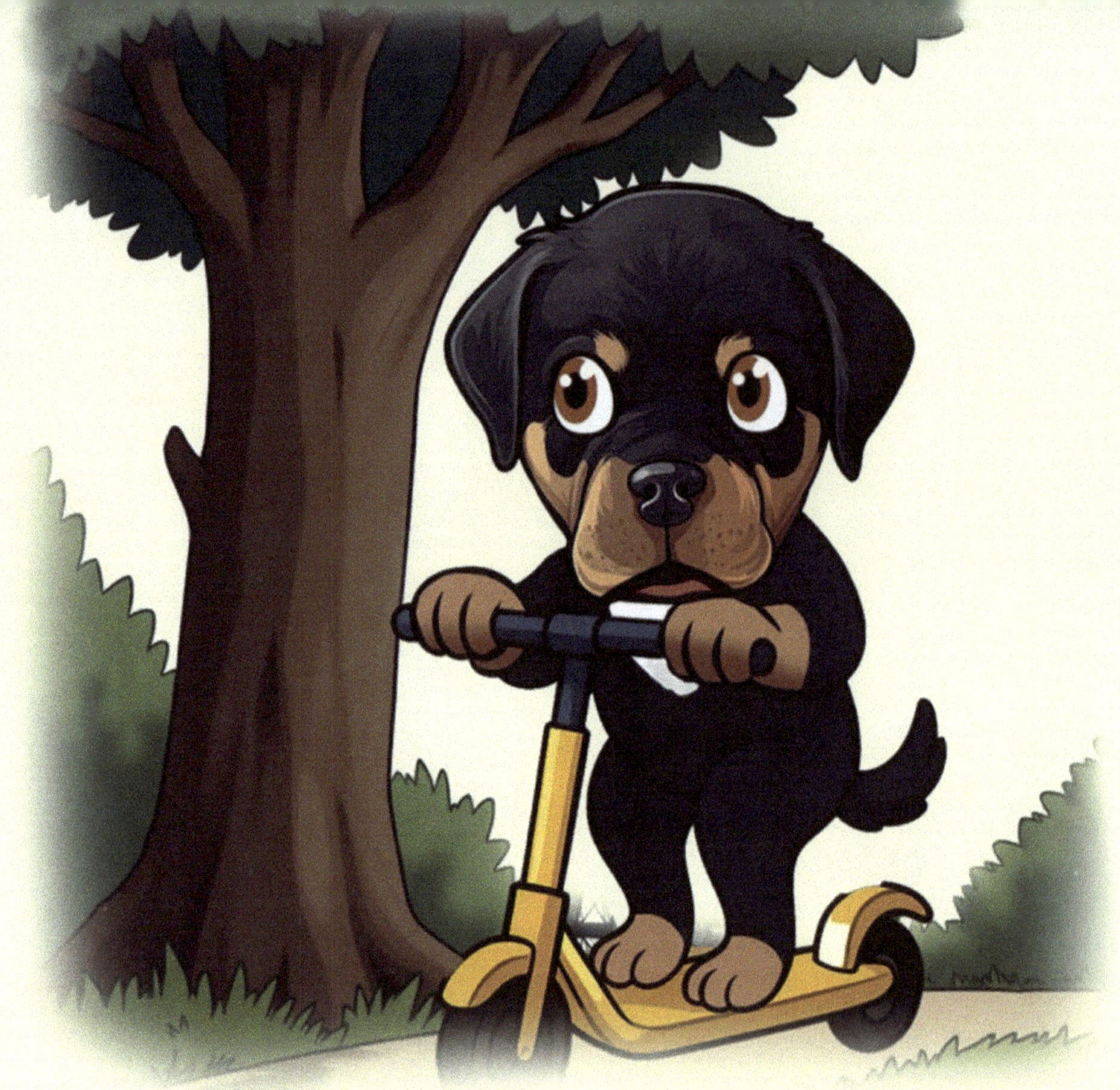

I was so busy thinking about those bullies on the way home that I nearly ran into a tree! I scared myself so bad I had to walk my scooter the rest of the way home!!

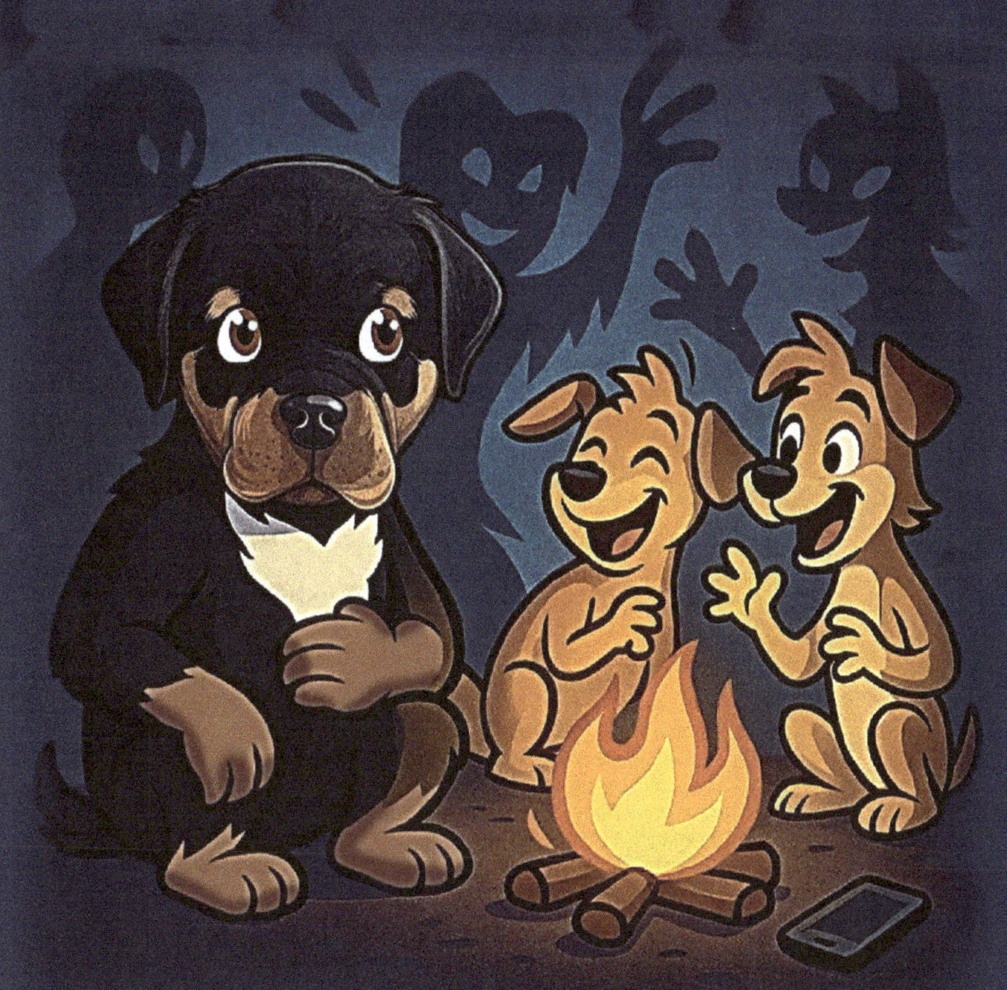

Since it was Friday, I got to have a sleepover at Kevin's house that night. The only problem was, all the other kids started telling ghost stories before bedtime. My stomach started to hurt, and I told Kevin that I needed to call my mom so she could come pick me up. I was too scared to stay all night.

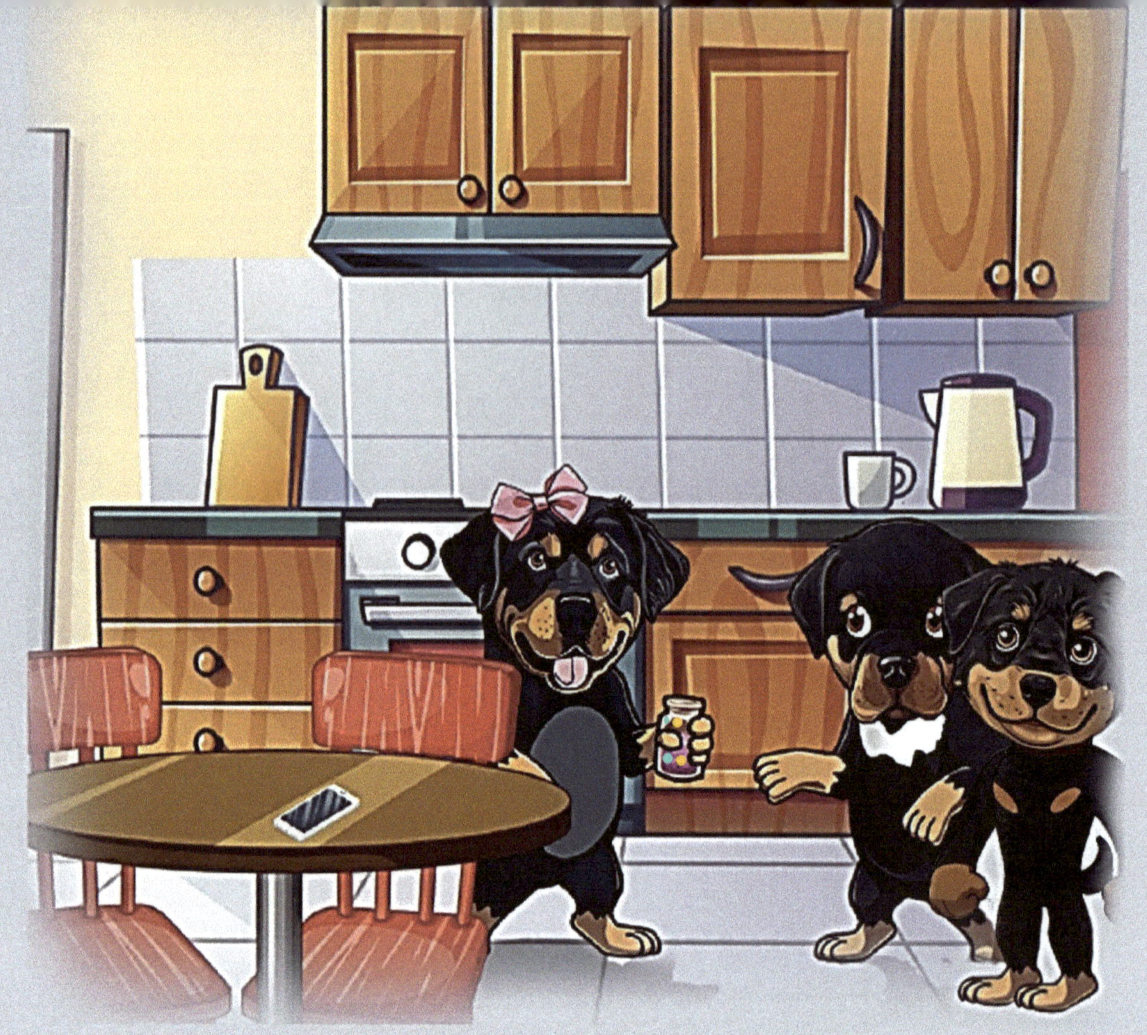

I was just about to call when Kevin's older sister, Angie, walked in. "What's up Simon?" she asked. "He's too nervous to stay over," Kevin answered for me. Angie looked at me sadly, then started walking around the kitchen opening and closing cabinets and drawers, collecting things as she went. She popped her gum loudly.

“I know what you’re going through,” she said. “I get anxious too.” “Really?” I asked. “Yep. And I’m going to show you some tricks to help you overcome that anxiety so you can do the things you want to do.” Angie brought a funnel, a spoon, and a bottle with water in it over to the kitchen table. “I’ll be right back,” she said, and disappeared down the hall to her bedroom. Soon Angie was back with a small jar of rainbow glitter. “What’s that for?” I asked. “Come sit down and I’ll show you,” she said. “Kevin, maybe you should go check on your other friends.” Kevin smiled and walked away.

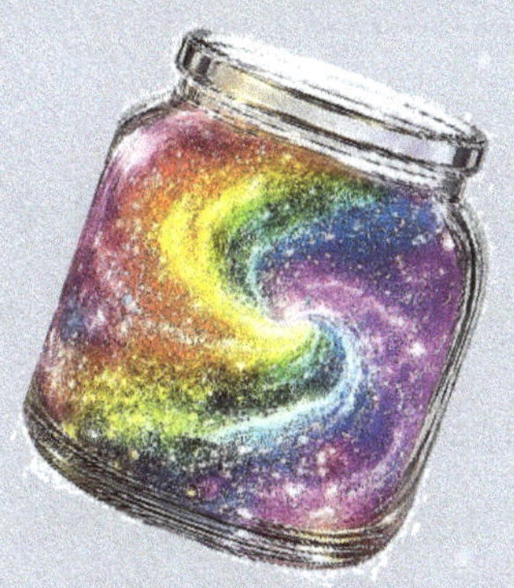

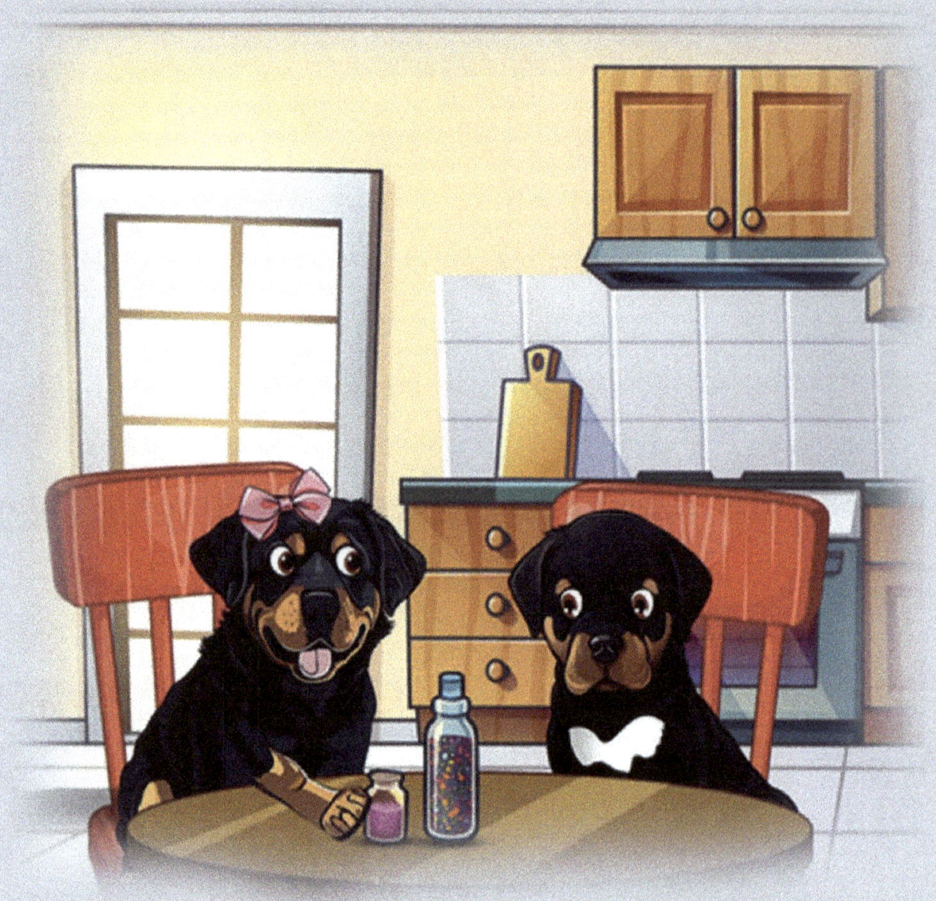

Alone in the kitchen, Angie and I sat at the table. “Let’s start by adding some glitter for every time you felt anxious today,” she said. I gave her a questioning look and waited. “Trust me?” she asked. “Okay,” I said.

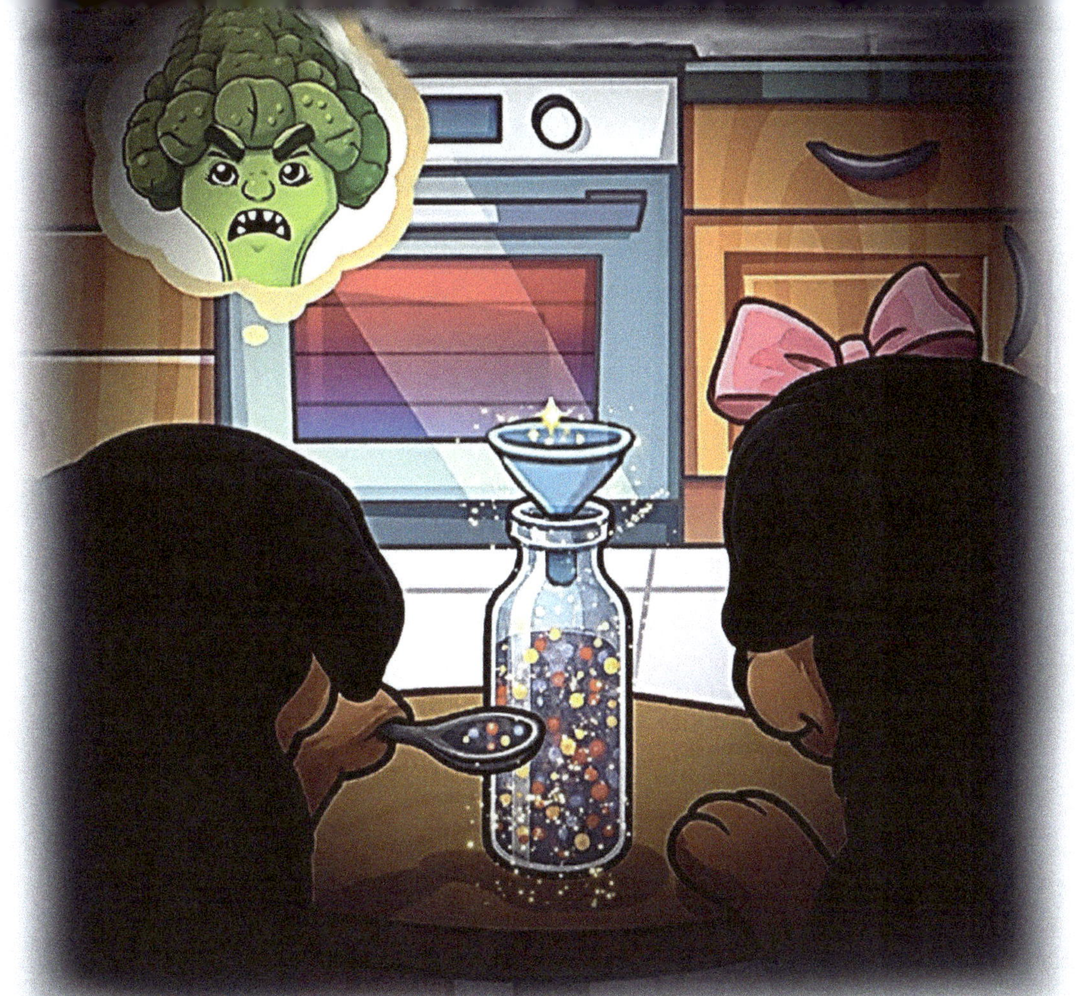

I picked up the spoon and scooped up some glitter from the jar. “I had a bad dream about a giant broccoli chasing me.” I dropped the glitter into the funnel and watched it pour into the water out the bottom end. “Kevin said there was a fire alarm at your school today,” Angie added. “I couldn’t tell if it was real!” I exclaimed and added another spoonful.

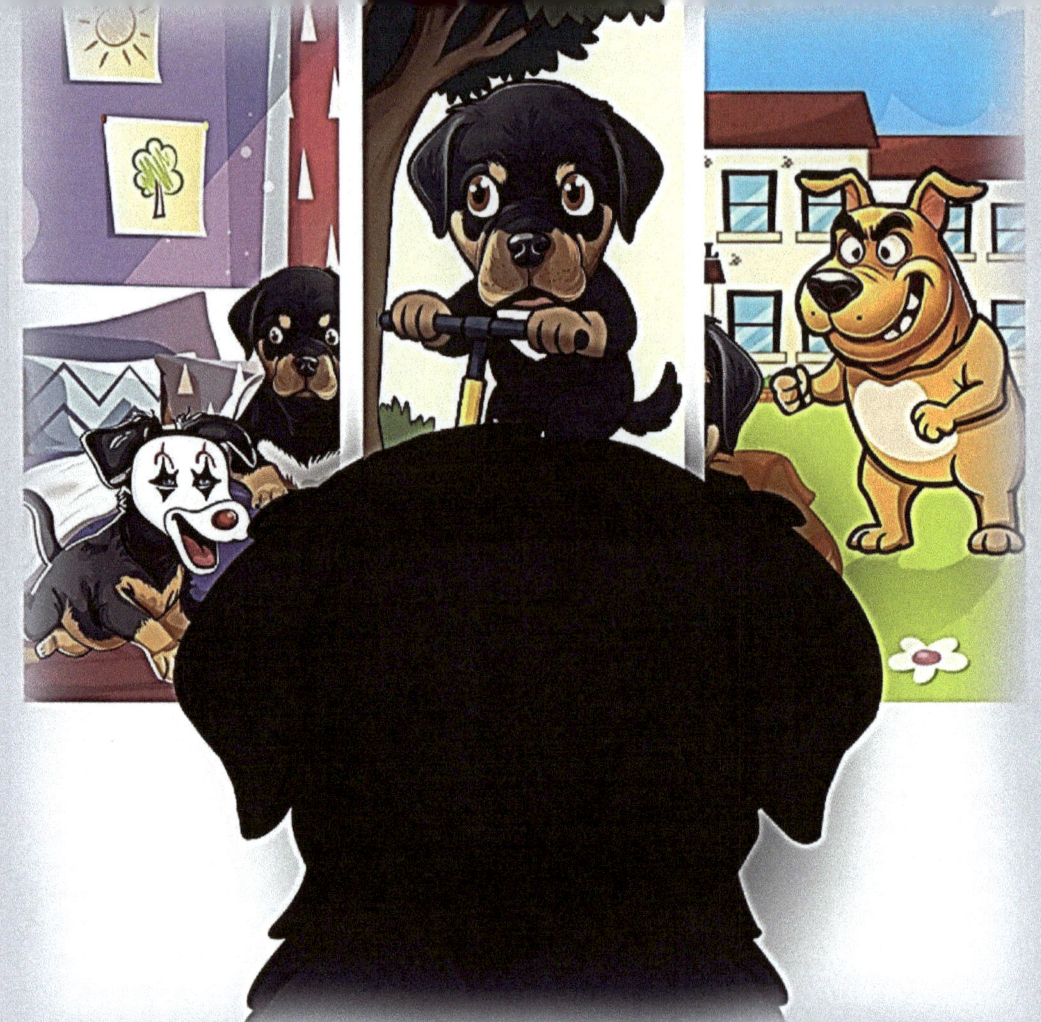

“What else ya got?” asked Angie. “My brother jumped out and scared me wearing a scary mask,” I said, dipping my spoon into the jar and adding more glitter to the water. “Anything else?” asked Angie. “Right before math class, I remembered we had a test and it was worth like half our grade,” I said, pouring another spoonful of glitter through the funnel.

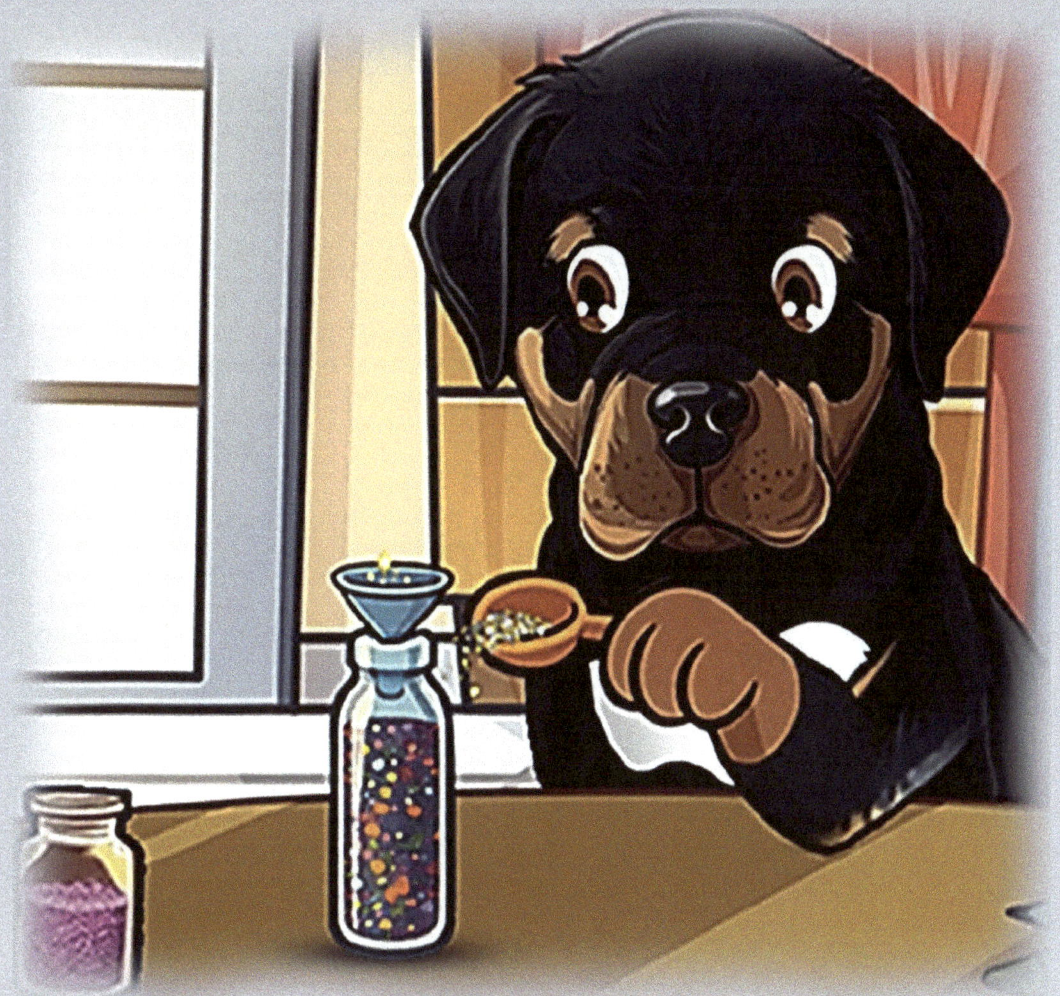

“Then I got distracted on my way home from school and almost hit a tree with my scooter,” I dumped some more glitter into the bottle. “Ouch,” said Angie. “And then everyone here was telling scary ghost stories, and it was just too much,” I mumbled adding the last spoonful of glitter to the water. “All done?” Angie asked. I nodded shamefully. “There’s nothing to be ashamed of. That sounds like a really rough day.”

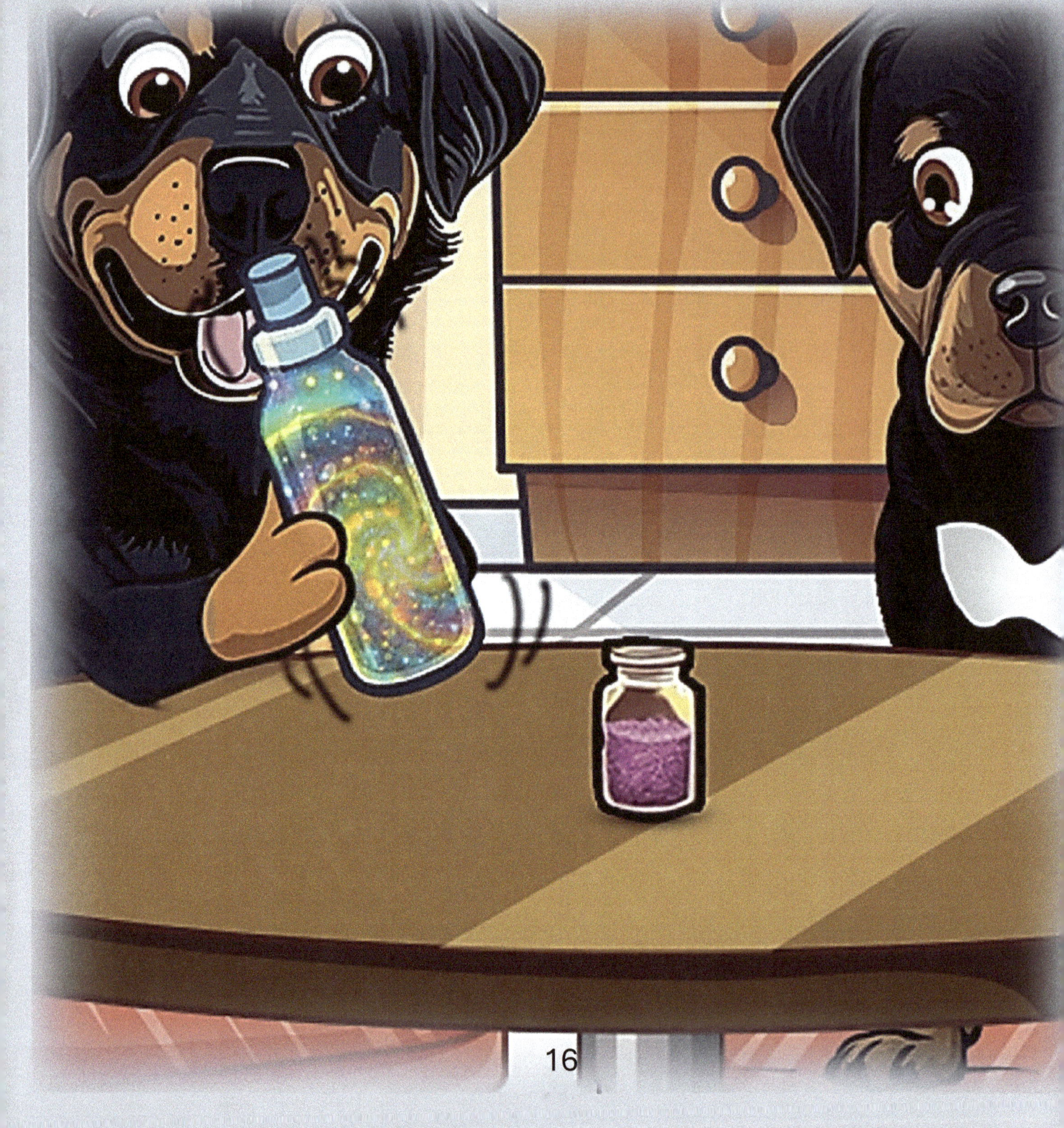

Angie put the lid on the bottle and shook it so that the glitter swirled wildly. “When I feel anxious, I shake up my thought bottle and then just sit and watch while the glitter settles. By the time the water is clear, my mind is too,” Angie explained. I gave her the side eye. I wasn’t buying it. “Trust me?” she asked. “Okay,” I said. I sat quietly and watched as the glitter fell, piece by piece, slowly to the bottom of the bottle. “Hey, it worked!” I said. “Cool right?” said Angie. “Can I keep that bottle?” I asked. “Of course!” Angie said. “I have one more thing I want to show you.”

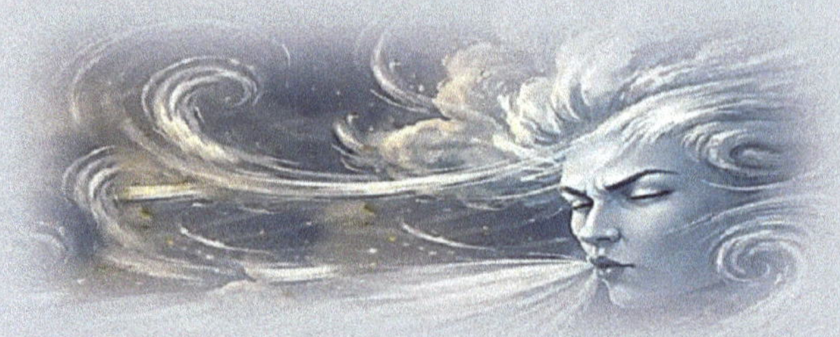

Still sitting at the kitchen table, Angie turned slightly to face me. “Make sure you’re comfortable, close your eyes, then put one paw on your belly, and the other paw in your lap,” followed Angie’s instructions. “Good,” she encouraged. “First take a normal breath. See how your chest moves?” “Yeah,” I said. “Now take a deep breath and try to move your paw on your belly instead,” Angie instructed me. I took a deep breath and focused on making my belly push my paw. “Take slow, deep breaths,” Angie said. As I did, I felt a sensation of calm come over my entire body. I closed my eyes and focused on just my breathing. All the worries of the day fell away. All the muscles in my body relaxed. I finally felt peaceful. When I opened my eyes, Angie was looking at me expectantly. “How do you feel?” she asked. “So relaxed,” I said. “I can’t even believe it.”

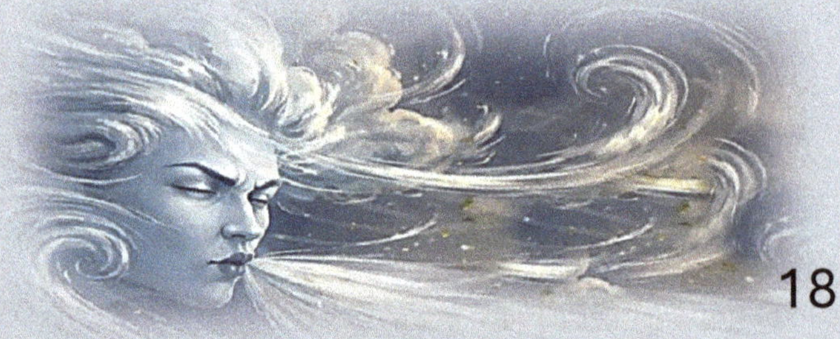

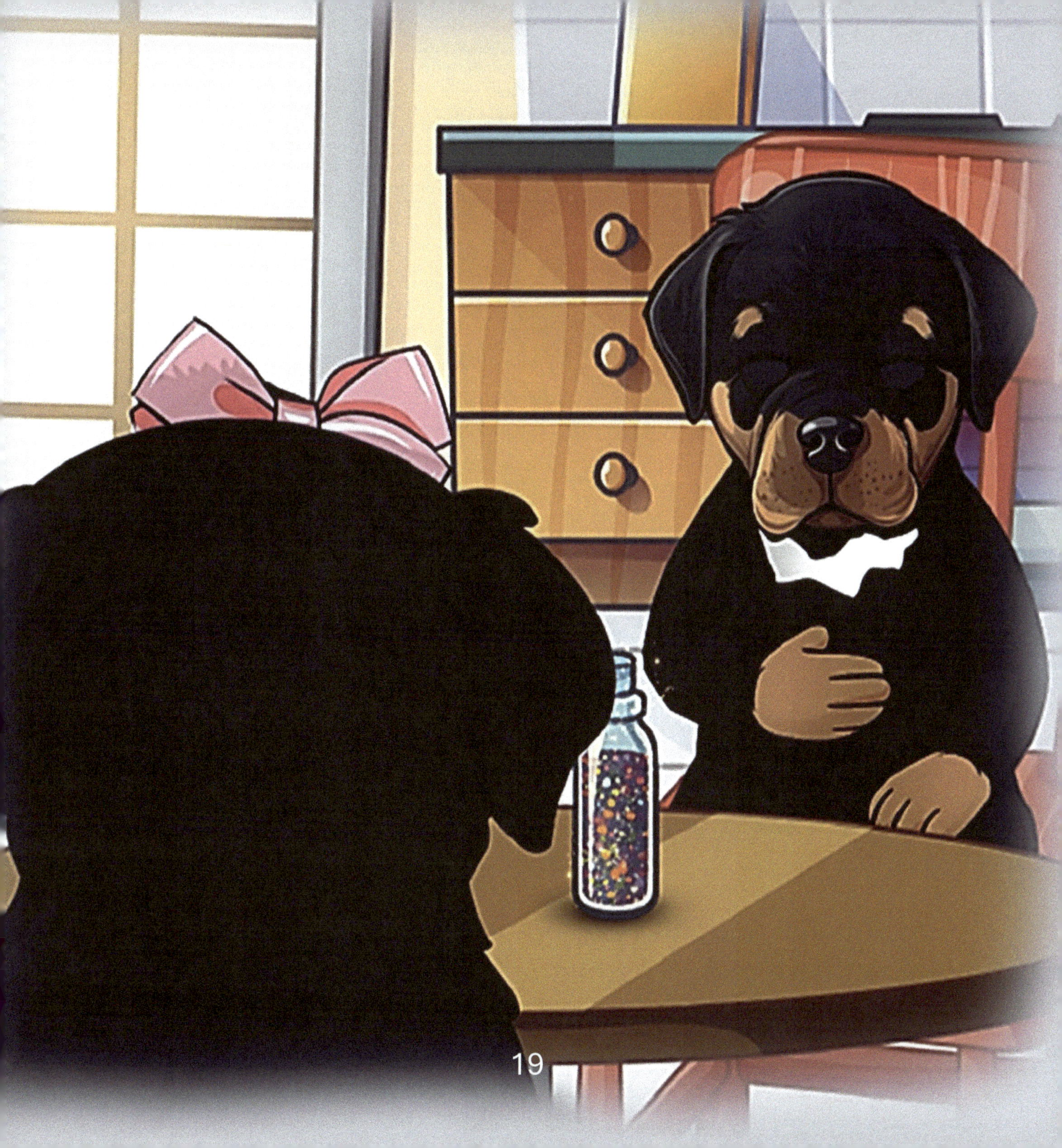

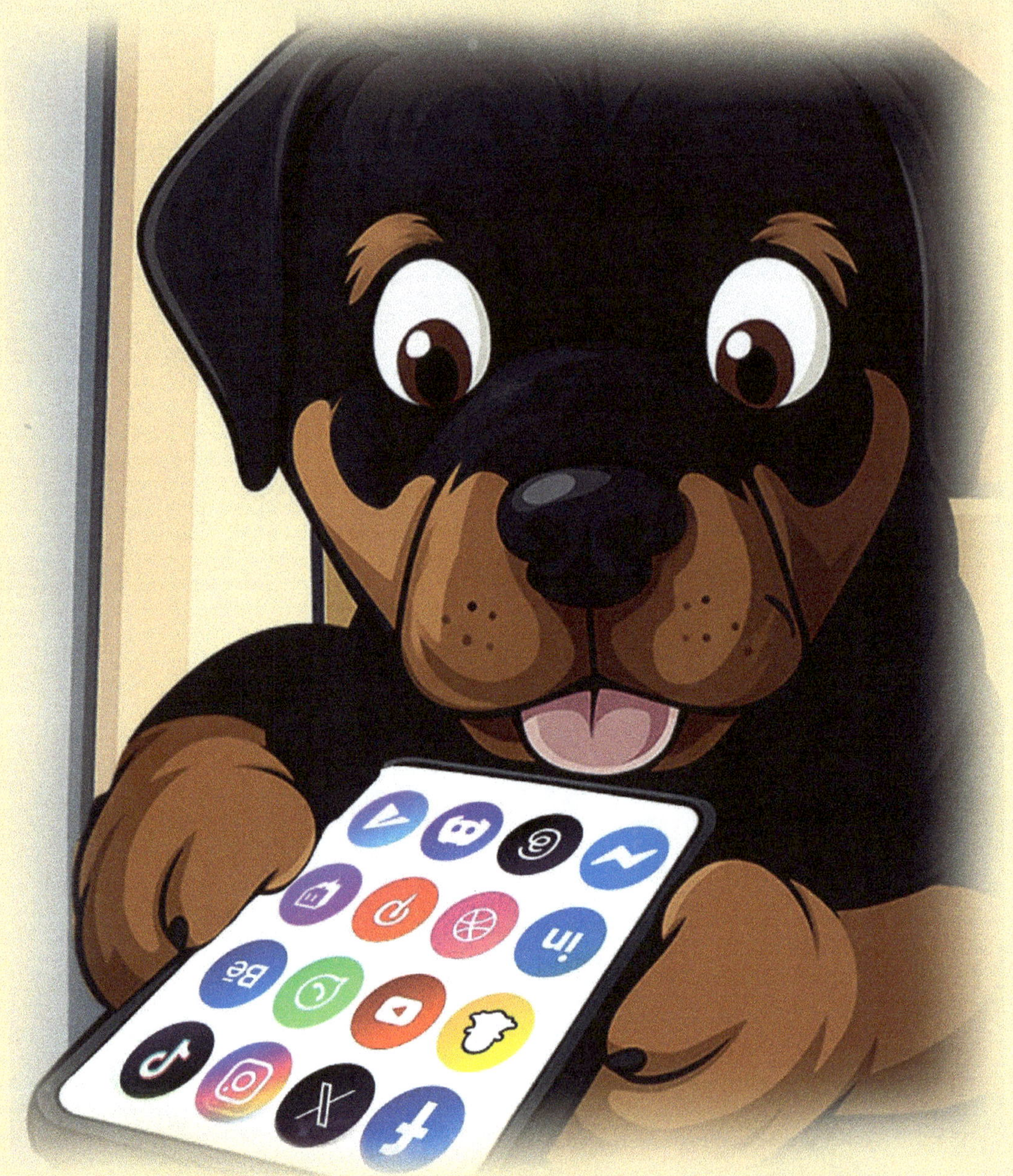

**“Do you still need to call your mom?” Angie asked. “Nah, I think I’ll be okay,” I smiled. “Thanks anyway.”**

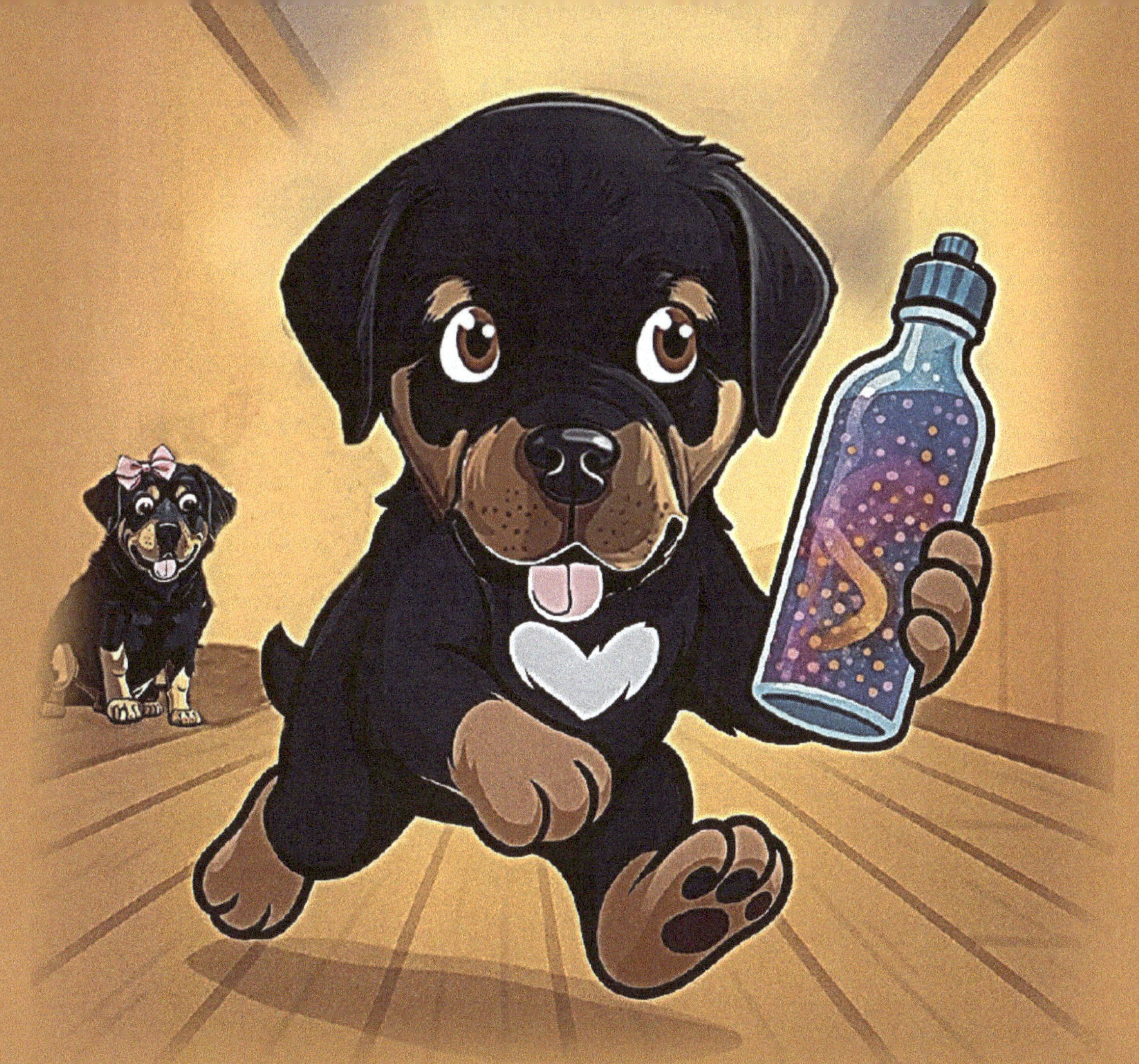

I grabbed my thought bottle and started to walk away. I stopped and turned around, and Angie looked surprised. “Thank you,” I said, “for everything.” “No problem,” Angie smiled. I turned and ran down the hallway to join my friends.

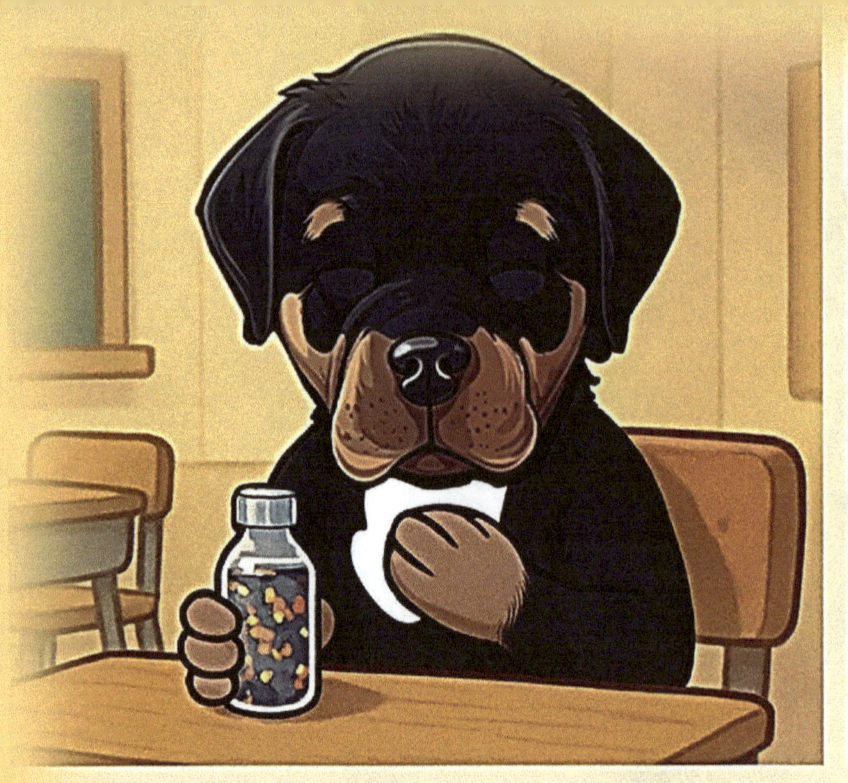
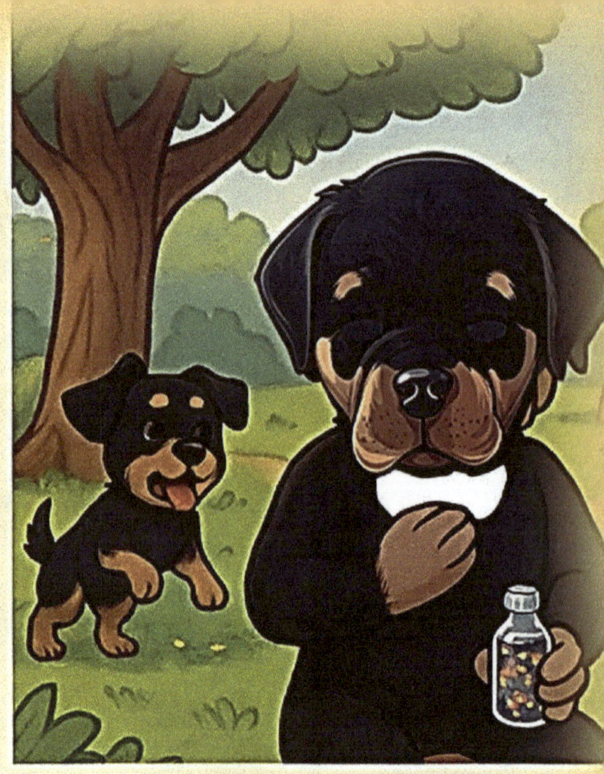
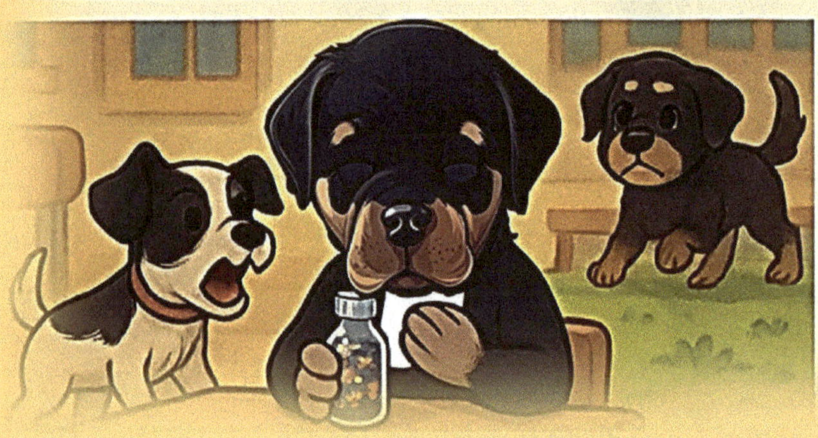
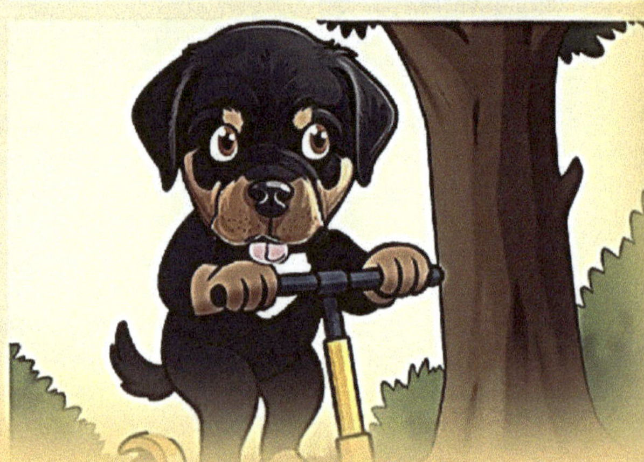

Now I use my thought bottle and my belly breathing whenever I feel anxious. Sometimes I use it when I know I might feel anxious, and it really helps me a lot.

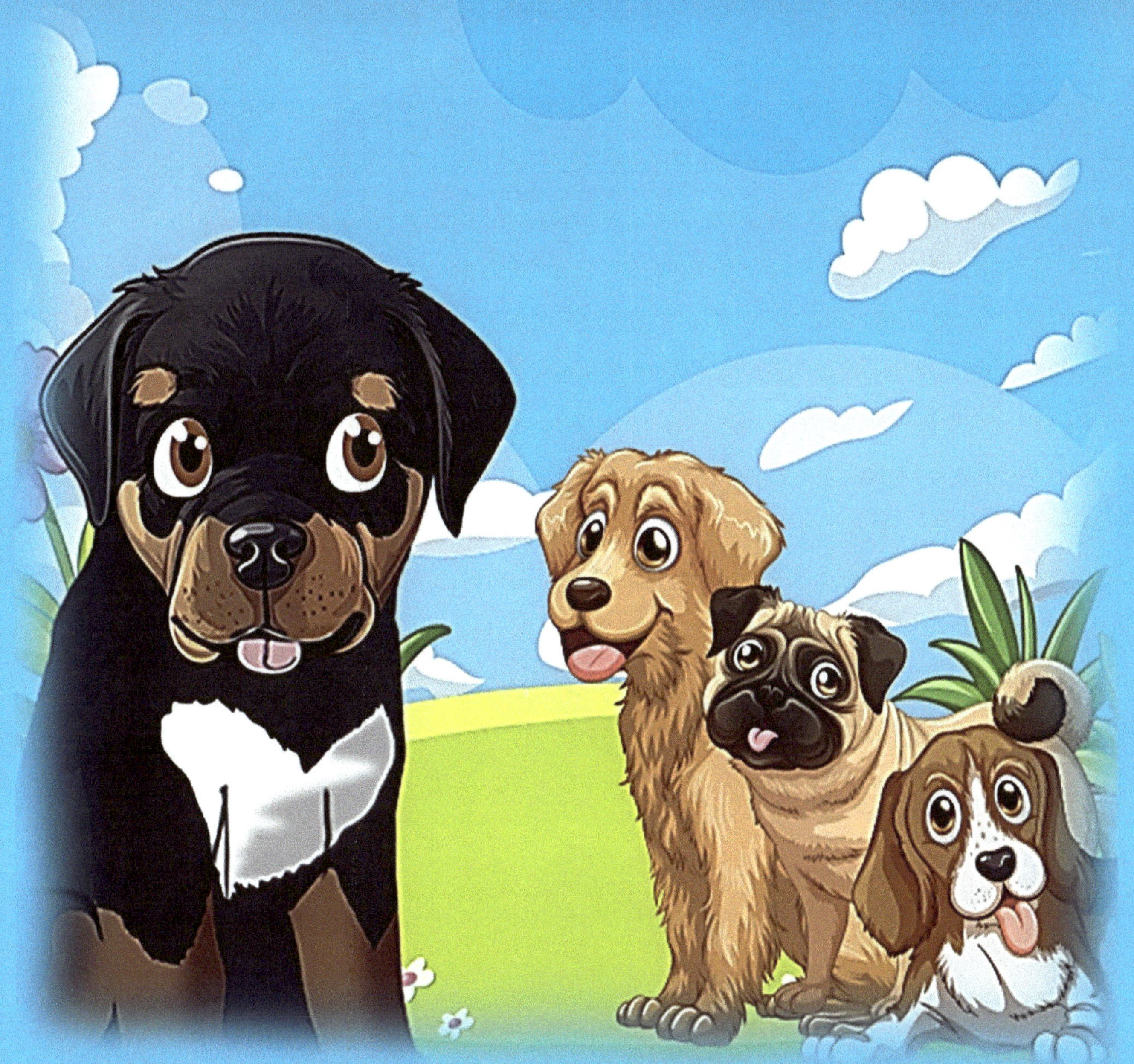

The best part is, I know I can handle things that happen to me, and that is the greatest feeling ever.

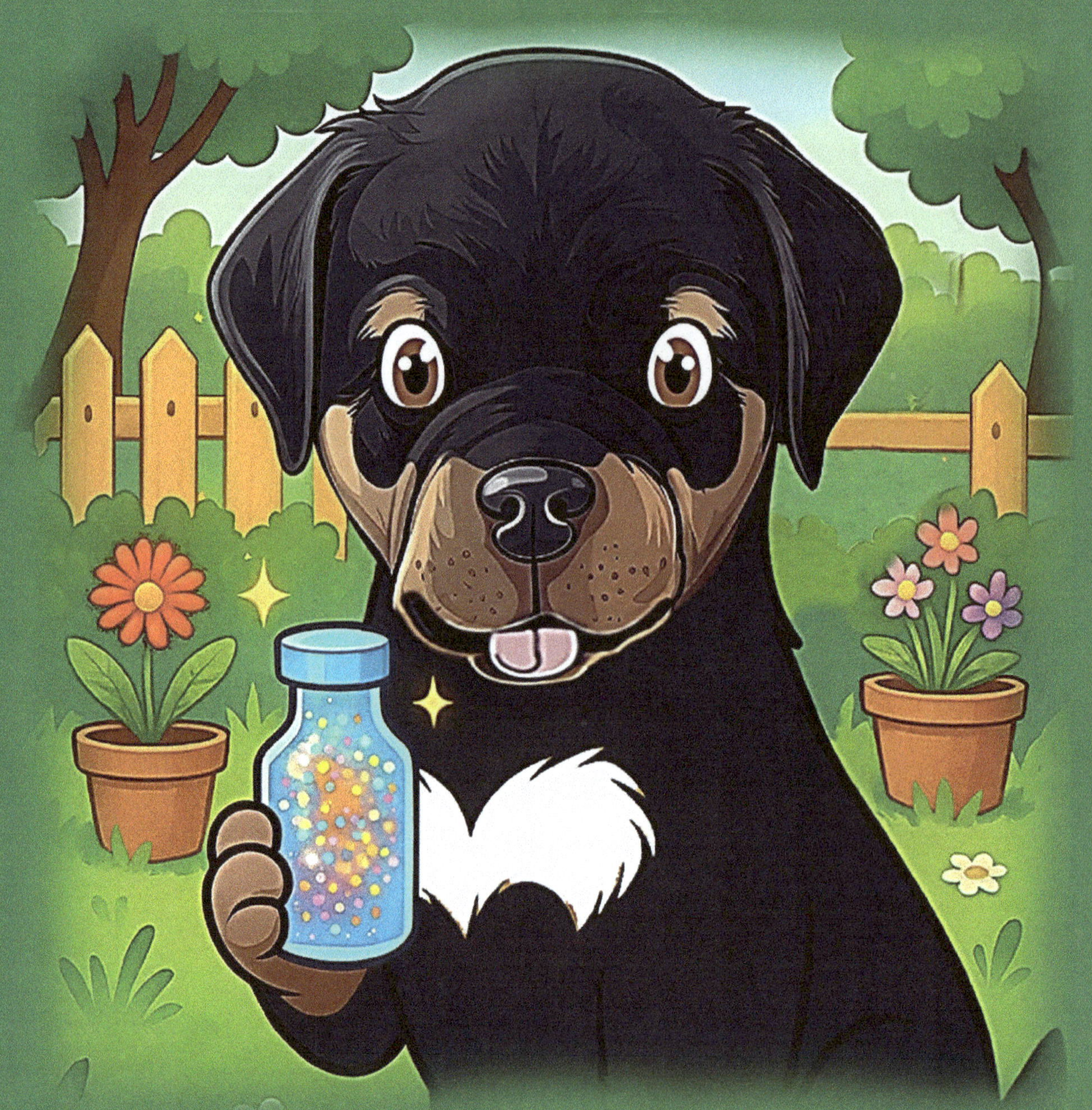

# The End

# Appendix

## How to Make a Thought Bottle

**What you will need:**

Clear plastic bottle, with lid (approx. 16 oz)

Glitter (I think fine works best, but it's really up to you)

Light Karo syrup (this keeps the glitter afloat in the water longer)

Liquid dish soap (just a drop - keeps the glitter from sticking together!)

Warm water (cold water and Karo syrup won't mix together)

Food coloring (to color the water; optional)

Super glue (to glue the lid on the bottle!)

---

**Directions:**

1. Put a drop of liquid dish soap in the bottom of the empty bottle.
2. Pour desired amount of glitter into the bottle.
3. Fill bottle approximately 1/3 full with light Karo syrup.
4. Add a drop or two of your food coloring (if applicable).
5. Fill the bottle the rest of the way full with warm water.
6. Apply super glue to the threads inside the lid, then screw the lid on tight.
7. Shake, shake, shake!

# Belly Breathing

1. Place one hand on your belly, just above your belly button.
2. Breathe normally. Notice how your chest moves.
3. Take a deep breath in through your nose, and at the same time, push your hand forward with your belly.
4. Breathe out slowly through your mouth.
5. Repeat as needed.

## National Child Anxiety Resources

- The Kids Mental Health Foundation (https://www.kidsmentalhealthfoundation.org/mental-health-resources/anxiety)
- American Academy of Child and Adolescent Psychiatry (https://www.aacap.org/aacap/Families_and_Youth/Resource_Centers/Anxiety_Disorder_Resource_Center/Home.aspx)
- Child Mind Institute (https://childmind.org/topics/anxiety/)
- National Institute of Mental Health (https://www.nimh.nih.gov/health/topics/anxiety-disorders)

# National Crisis Resources

- National Suicide and Crisis Lifeline (988)
- National Hotline For Mental Health Crises and Suicide Prevention (800-273-TALK (8255))
- Crisis Text Line (Text HOME to 741741)
- Veterans Crisis Line (988, then press 1 or Text 838255)
- National Child Abuse Hotline (800) 422-4453

www.ingramcontent.com/pod-product-compliance
Lightning Source LLC
LaVergne TN
LVHW060643110826
845147LV00018B/1035

* 9 7 9 8 2 1 8 8 8 4 8 0 2 *